Elephant in the Room

Plus Size. Plus Life.
Plus Experience …

—

… My Way!

© 2017 S Shelby

All rights reserved.

**Library of Congress Control Number: 2018934801
Elephant In The Room, Maryland Heights, MO**

ISBN: 0-692-97672-8

ISBN 13: **978-0-692-97672-2**

Published by Sharita Shelby

For more information Sharita Shelby and Elephant in the Room visit, www. eitr-sshelby.com

ELEPHANT IN THE ROOM

Introduction

Let's tackle this elephant! I know most books typically explain a deep-rooted need for the inspiration of their words, but mine is simple. I have spent my life, from nine years old to now, as a "plus-size" woman. Listen to my thoughts about this experience. I will use many different words to describe being a woman of weight, and my word choice is definitely intentional because words and labels have power. Plus-size ladies, know that someone can completely relate to you, your stories, your laughs, and your fears. Those of you who have no clue, I want you to know that weight is not just a physical attribute but a lifestyle and experience that you probably had no clue existed. So now, just maybe you won't think of the big girls differently, or at least, since this book exists, you will be able to understand our plight better. I can't say I have been bullied, had low self-esteem per se, or inadequacy, so I can't address that- sorry. Simply, I've had the journey of a girl who evolved into a woman who has had to embrace a full-figured lifestyle. After the inception of my book, I made the decision for a lifestyle change that allowed my weight to reduce significantly, but I'm still plus size and still live this story every day. I am now on the larger side of the rack instead of the larger section of the store. The Elephant in the Room

ELEPHANT IN THE ROOM

(EITR) is a saying that describes a topic, a situation, or in some cases a person that people want to avoid or don't want to discuss. Being plus size can be the elephant, literally, but this book will put it all out there, and it won't be the elephant in this room!

I want to put out three messages with this book:

1. I want you to feel that our imperfections are our unique perfections. Beauty is in the eye of the beholder, and we have the power of the eye but sometimes the tongue of a beast. If we could see others as we want to be seen ourselves, then there would be no elephant in the room. The imperfection also known as weight is still our unique perfection.

2. I want you to be aware of the journey of women and especially plus-size women in the United States. This story of weight not only opens you up to the world's view but also challenges your own views. This is a topic I rarely have heard mentioned, but it is real, and I want to tackle this elephant.

3. I want to make you smile and laugh about my world, from my view. I want you to have a relatable moment, even if it's just one sentence. I want you to ride along with me in this journey of my purpose and my story.

ELEPHANT IN THE ROOM

Acknowledgements

I want to thank my parents and brother for never allowing my weight to be an excuse to limit me. I am thankful to my friends for allowing me to be just me, with them, at any size. To my "terrific three" line sisters, thanks for motivating me from vision to completion. To my God, I just want to thank you for the journey and this confidence that you put in my soul!

ELEPHANT IN THE ROOM

Table of Contents

Elephants 1–23

1. That Your Mother?!
2. Where It All Started
3. Genetics: The Fat Gene
4. Prom
5. Diets!
6. You Know Those Pants Don't Look Good on You!
7. My Pull…
8. Biggirlswithgoodcredit.com
9. What Was That?
10. Black Girls Don't Run
11. Spandex, All Spandex
12. These Ain't Your Mama's Rolls
13. Out to Eat
14. What's Been Eating Her?
15. Seat-Belt Extender
16. The Size of Adventure
17. Three Hundred and You're Done!
18. Hypochondriac
19. The Decision
20. Still Big: The Post Surgery Challenge
21. I Get an A for Acceptance
22. Looking to the Hills
23. I Come as One, but I Stand as Ten Thousand

ELEPHANT IN THE ROOM

Elephant 1

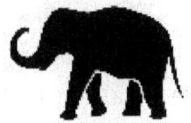

That Your Mother?

ELEPHANT IN THE ROOM

Yes, I'm sure when you read the title of this chapter you said, "Is that proper English?" Well, let's just say I borrowed it from my many Asian brothers and sisters who state this same line every time they encounter my mother and me while enjoying some girl time at the nail shop. "You so big; she so little," they would say. See, my mother is about five feet five and used to wear a size 4 dress. She has aged well, might I add. She is now about an 8. However, compared to me, one might envision the comparison between the elephant and the mouse, or King Kong and that little woman he holds in his hand. I say this because I stand almost six feet tall and more than 300 pounds. Those people, unaware of how it made me feel, often made comments like this not just privately between my mother and I, but in front of others, and at times in front of everyone in Kansas City who chose to get her nails done that day. At these moments, I was more embarrassed than hurt because they didn't know me and really were just trying to spark up conversation. Little did they know that this could play on my insecurity of knowing I looked different than my mother. I looked like my dad, who they never saw and somewhat discounted by emphasizing the size difference. Because of these types of incidents, I couldn't help but to begin to explore my true feelings of others discussing my weight.

The reason others' comments weren't so hurtful was that the elephant was welcome in the room at my house, and often discussed. I am taller and bigger than both my parents and my brother who was a Rose Bowl championship football player and now a college football coach. I can even remember my father saying on multiple occasions, "If we could have just switched the size of the two of you, we could have really made some money," meaning that if my brother were my size and height, he would have been an NFL player.

One thing that you will learn about my family is that there is not too much that won't be said. So, if you are sensitive, this is not the family for you. I can say that we are not intentionally offensive, just open to sharing our thoughts and feelings freely without much consideration for the feelings of others. That's normal, right? We love each other, and therefore the feedback was sacred because it was from the people that love you the most. With this as my foundation, I can say that outwardly I'm not the most sensitive person. There are few things that can get right to the core of me. Comments made by general observation

ELEPHANT IN THE ROOM

don't tend to bother me because I realize that typically they are subjective. They don't hold much merit for me. Three things bother me: talking about my family, throwing it in my face that I ever needed to ask for your help, or making a full character judgment about me. If you say one of those things, then *bam*—you have gotten to me.

I will be beyond bothered, and you or anyone that tries me can be one second away from seeing an entirely different me!

In my family, I can say that typically things stated wouldn't be outright mean; the words definitely weren't lined with sugar but could be seen by others as served as a side of s#@!. For example, in our family, I never heard I was beautiful. But if I wore something that looked good or fit well, my dad would say, "You should have gotten two of those," implying I looked good. That was my sugar, but not saying I was beautiful ever could be seen as kinda crappy.

My mother did the best she could with me, even though she didn't know what to do with this child in the sixth grade who was already fitting into her clothes. How do you clothe a daughter in the plus-size section when you have never been to that side of the store? How do you handle her chubbiness or introducing a diet when you have never been on one? What do you do with this child who is so different from you? She was a determined mother, and I knew my size was different. So, I had been to Slim for Life, a local Weight Watchers–type program, wrapped in some type of mummy outfit to lose inches and on the cabbage diet all before the age of seventeen! The journey of weight loss began early, often like learning how to ride a bicycle. When you are just coming off the training wheels, you ride with all confidence, like joining Weight Watchers, but until you have fallen to the ground—your diet fails—you realize it's not that easy. You really must learn to ride and stay on, like making a lifestyle change instead of participating in crash diets. Despite my early dieting efforts, this fluffy body still had to be clothed.

My mother insisted that I wear nice clothes. I probably was dressed better than most thirty-nine-year-old women. My mother was not okay with thin material, cheap zippers, unlined pants, not having proper undergarments, or clothes that would shrink in the wash. So, she paid for quality and insisted that I would, too. At the time clothes that were bigger tended to be for adult women. I remember standing in the Ups and Downs which is like the current New

ELEPHANT IN THE ROOM

York and Company, and my mother bringing me to the counter, saying, "What do you have to fit her?"

The lady looked me up and down like a five-legged puppy just to see what I needed. I was bigger than the average girl and younger than the average plus-size woman. Then it happened—I was like an elephant in the middle of the room. Sadly, this resulted in a day in the store trying on junior's clothes that were tight and short and adult women's clothes that made me look forty. Needless to say, we did walk out with a few basics, but a twelve-year-old's wardrobe was not one of them.

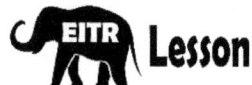 **Lesson**

People will say anything! But when they do, you have to decide how you are going to take in the information because their words and your young age can turn into the conscience of your life. What do you want to hear in the back of your mind? You must decide.

Elephant 2

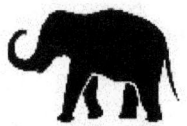

Where It All Started

ELEPHANT IN THE ROOM

My Entrance

I was born on a beautiful summer day in August 1979. My parents had been married for seven years, and after several attempts and miscarriages, there I was, but of course not without taking everything out of my mother. My mother lost so much blood that they weren't sure if she was going to make it. So, I guess even my entrance into this world was "big." Being that my parents waited so long in anticipation of having a child, I can say my life was intentional from its inception, and just how so, would be much clearer later in life. Every step of my journey would lead me to who I would become.

My Weird Relationship

Growing up there were always some small areas of contention between my mom and me. My acceptance of myself and my size began when I had to figure out me and my place in this world on my own. I equated the years of awkwardness between my mom and I to the fact that she was used to having all of my dad's time and attention to herself, and then here comes this little girl who is now the apple of his eye. She wouldn't intentionally withhold emotion or guidance, but she was just not sure how to raise a girl, one that was so different from herself. This is

ELEPHANT IN THE ROOM

only theory based on no facts, but I needed to create this in my world for our strained relationship to make sense to me. All I wanted was for my mom to dote on me, be the Girl Scout leader, cook fabulous home-cooked meals, not eat out so much, paint nails together, and just be present. I have never even said these things out loud to myself until now. But instead I was just a daughter on a mission with my mother, who was trying to figure out just what to do with me.

I remember one time her verbalizing her discomfort to her friends: "Rita has gained weight, and I just don't know what to do with her. "One of her friends suggested putting me in dance. As different friends weighed in on the solution of what she should do with her fat daughter, I just looked at them. I remember being embarrassed. Some of my odd embarrassments to this day started out with these few life-changing moments of standing in front of people and having them provide unsolicited feedback about me—at least not solicited by me.

My Schooling

I went to private school most of my life. I always had friends and was in the "in crowd." I was best friends with the "grownest" little woman most had known. She was smart beyond her years and was never afraid to say what was on her mind, from the age of six to today. She was my best friend from first grade until high school and still is one of my best friends to this day. She was the most popular and the ring leader of most things, and I was her best friend. She was the only person with whom I could go places, and hers was the only house where I could spend the night. Luckily my best friend looked kind of like me: brown skin like me, normal-girl height like me, and a fluffy girl like me. I never had to worry about trying to fit in with her. She was my spoiled friend who got everything she wanted, who had parents that would move heaven and earth to make her happy. And, what I can say? As her friend, I reaped the benefits, too! There was no place her dad wouldn't drive us or anything we wanted that he wouldn't bend backward to do for us. We would go all day and hang out and eat, but if we wanted an Icee from Seven-Eleven at midnight, he would leave immediately to address our needs, even if it meant driving to the hood and dodging a bullet to get a cherry-and-blue mixed Icee. He was like my dad, and he instilled princess qualities in both of us early.

ELEPHANT IN THE ROOM

Having this friendship of parallel values and similar looks helped to form me and validated that my world was consistent with my bestie's. So, I was never forced to consider what was consistent with most girls my age.

My Bestie

Having this friend eliminated most of my troubles from the first to twelfth grade because I had my place. Our friendship was never tested or needed any outline early on because we were from similar worlds. We wore the same size, shopped at the same stores, had similar parental environments, and shared many of the same values. Even as we began to have years apart at different schools, our friendship was natural, uncomplicated and perfect for me. I was accepted by her and other school-age peers. Having a great relationship with my dad and having positive interaction with her dad, I was taught very young to embrace my inner princess and require respect.

My Change

Things started to change for me slightly. Around the fourth grade, I began to gain weight. It probably was only about fifteen pounds, but it was a noticeable difference in my school pictures the next two years.

ELEPHANT IN THE ROOM

The counselor in me equates it to a time where things changed for me. I attended a new school, got new friends, and my mom returned to college. My dad began to spend a lot of time with us. Amid this change, I began my relationship with food.

I had always been close with my dad. He had always done more than his fair share in our daily routine due to the flexibility of being an entrepreneur. Now, we spent any time not in school with him. He always made a great breakfast, but we began the era of microwaving Banquet frozen dinners and throwing a pot pie in the oven. Around this time, I remember cleaning up the kitchen at night and eating the leftover food. It was dark. I was alone. My family had retreated to their rooms, and there I was with the food. I can't say for certain how this started, but I certainly can understand the realities of it now. When you begin an unhealthy relationship with food, it is because it fills something within you. The voids of my mother's absence, the change in school, and missing my old friends was now a void that I needed to fill. Food is consistent and never disappoints. When I eat a cookie to this day, it tastes the same. It never disappoints! It's always consistent, unlike people, schools, or even life. I remember wanting to clean the dishes just so I could eat more. This is when

ELEPHANT IN THE ROOM

I started gaining weight. I was becoming what the world would call heavy, a little bigger than most kids, overweight, obese and my favorite - I just didn't grow out of my baby fat.

My Struggle

In these early years, I knew that I began to have unsure thoughts of who I was and how I fit into my family. I had to be approximately nine years old around the time of my weight gain. Due to a growing distant relationship with my mom and what seemed to be a consistent level of ill will toward me for some reason I could never explain, it was the first time that my thoughts started to take form and supersede just being present. I began to wonder about fitting in my family and began to form thoughts in my head to rationalize my feelings in my heart. My first theory of my awkwardness with my mom was that I wasn't my mom's biological child because I felt she had such disdain for me. Maybe I was adopted, and therefore her patience with me was short because she was just learning to accept me. After digging through old pictures and keepsakes, I was unable to draw any strong conclusions for this theory. So that left me with a thought that maybe I just wasn't meant to be here, on earth. I had thoughts of suicide. I didn't really have a plan or means, but I thought maybe I should just kill myself. Thinking back, I'm not even sure how I knew about suicide or what would make me have such a dark thought, but I did. I even went as far as telling my dad I wanted to kill myself because I just couldn't understand why we didn't seem to gel like other mothers and daughters. All I remember is him saying, "Don't you ever let somebody make you feel that way and have that kind of power over your life! Nobody! Not even your mother!" That was my two minutes of daddy therapy that changed my life forever. Power that I had given to someone else I realized was mine. I would take that knowledge into forever because it was my dragon slayer in situations where I felt, awkward, different or any small moments of inadequacy.

ELEPHANT IN THE ROOM

My Esteem

Despite these early moments, I developed a healthy self-esteem. I was a cheerleader, ran track (ha!), had friends, was very involved with church, and enjoyed my life. I didn't want for anything, and I grew up with a strong sense of family. Almost every Sunday we went over to my grandmother's house for Sunday dinners, and the village had their turn in my life. We spent time with both sides of my family. By the time I entered high school, I had decided that I wanted to be cute, wear fashionable clothes, use my voice, and be my own "diva." Besides, I was smart and developed a good self-esteem. I was always selected for leadership roles in school, and I had strong village to groom my esteem into the lady I would later become.

Beyond the veil of obesity, we generally had a happy family. Both my parents were hard workers, and my mom was a go-getter in my eyes. I even remember when I was asked to talk about my mom for a presentation in school. All I remember saying was that she was a career mom. I didn't have any funny bake-sale stories or experiences playing dolls. However, I knew she worked hard, and we didn't want for anything. And most important I knew she loved me. She had a career and needed to take care of us. My dad was an entrepreneur of a club and sporting-goods store. I was front row seeing the commitment of making something work in an ever-changing world. From being in the beauty shop or out and about, I was subject to hearing people weigh in on the family business and all the people that worked for us. I suppose it built resilience, but most important it built awareness and the need to know the truth about where I came from and how I would live my truth. It was clear that if I did not make my claims on my world, the community would.

 **Lesson**

Your childhood begins the blueprint of your life. It doesn't guarantee the structure, but it does secure the foundation.

Elephant 3

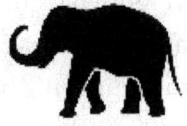

Genetics: The Fat Gene

ELEPHANT IN THE ROOM

I've been heavy since the fourth grade. All of a sudden, I had cheeks and of course a new Jheri curl, a hair fad of the 80's. Basically, I was a cute and chubby little boy. For a Jheri curl, you must cut off all the hair straightened by a relaxer. I lost several inches and ended up with a curly afro. I was having a hair evolution, and my weight was going through one, too. Over the years all I heard was that I looked just like my daddy, and of course it's because he is my heavy parent. So even though many of my facial features were like my mom, I was my dad's twin. People even called me by my last name just because that side of my family carried a little more weight. I guess that is just how it goes. Based on our features and behaviors, people decide which side of the family we all favor. For many of us, it's not just a fat gene. It's just whatever you do or don't do that is inherent to one side of your family, like:

"Girl he is always in trouble! He gets that from his daddy."

"I don't know why he is so short. Well, his mom's side is short!"

We all just rush to categorize people, and all that is bad or unsure gets thrown to the other side of the family. I guess I will just take the paternal-side fat gene and make it look good! At least that's what I thought.

Over the years one thing I heard about obesity was that it is genetic. Like a real, live fat gene. Now, who can combat that? That was a great reason that I couldn't control my weight, and that explained everything, right? It made perfect sense to me in the long list as to why my weight was not my fault. It reminds me of a funny story, but not so funny, when my mom, the thin one, had to get double bypass heart surgery.

The doctor wanted to talk to all of us about her surgery, her new diet, and our family risk factors of heart disease. When the doctor was ready to speak to us, I had left the hospital, of course, to go eat. When I got back, my brother and dad were in tears laughing so hard. My brother was bent over, and my dad was leaning back laughing as if they were watching Comedy Central. They told me when they walked in, the doctor said, "Where is that other one? The big one!"

Dad said, "Well, she went to eat!" smirking to himself.

ELEPHANT IN THE ROOM

"Well, she needs to be in here because she is at high risk for everything!" She went on to explain, considering all my genetic traits.

She looked at my brother and said, "You may be all right. You seem like you take good care of yourself, but that other one. She needs to be careful because she is at risk for all of these!" She pointed to the list of health risks.

Disease by disease she went through the list, and after each one she said, "The other one needs to be aware of this."

So, yes, it's been confirmed I have bad genes. I didn't even have to be present for a doctor to know that I was struggling with my genes, and they were going to affect me negatively one day. My mother has said this since I can remember, but this doctor's consultation was verification of this. My brother and dad thought it was so funny and me too, honestly. On the inside, I knew she was right, and the road ahead would be uphill.

Do I believe that there is a fat gene? Of course, I do! I know that exercise, diet and determination can help combat this. *But how unfair!* I've thought since my first diet, "Why did I have to get this gene and spend my whole existence focused on food choices, scales, large clothing and just the stigma of being a fat girl?" I'd think at times I wish I just had small lips, a shorter arm, or maybe something genetically inside where others would not have to see. This gene is honest, and it sure does come with a lot. To all the genetically thin women, I say enjoy, I guess. I mean, I know it must be a challenge to a have small chest, no hips, or a butt that doesn't fill out your pants, but hey, life is a tradeoff. At least you can walk into a store in the mall and shop for whatever you want! And, they say you will live longer. Wanna trade?

 **Lesson**

We don't get a choice in our genetic make-up, and it's all a matter of chance how the result of our gene pool will affect us. If you got the fat gene, first you have to accept it. You have to decide if you want to do anything about it, and then, you just gotta be the best version of your fluffy self.

Elephant 4

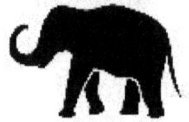

Prom

ELEPHANT IN THE ROOM

It's the day that all girls dream of. Quite honestly it is the virtual bridge to the dream wedding that you always envisioned. It's a sign that you finally have grown up. It is the only date that your parents preapprove. It's the bridge to womanhood and, if you're lucky, the night of your life. Used to be the night where virginity was taken. Across America, and, at Saint Teresa's Academy, a wonderful all-girls Catholic school, prom was a one-time event. We did not have two opportunities to get it right. It was your senior year, and that was it. For girls, it's the event that you plan for from Christmas break forward, and of course once spring break came, you were just moments away from the biggest night of your high school life. As a typical girl, I was trying to make sure I secured my date. Lucky for me, I already had a tentative boyfriend already ready. As the known planner I am, even at seventeen, I was making sure we had a limo, identified the location for dinner, set preprom arrival time, and planned after-party logistics. And due to my maturity, I guess—more like my desire to have the perfect night—I got my parents to allow all the couples to spend the night at our house. With all this anticipation and excitement, what could change the hopes of the senior prom? The daunting task of dress shopping!

Well, I will be honest. The mental preparation was much more difficult than the physical locating of the dress. I knew that even though it was 1997, most formal wear in a size 22 was made for ladies at least twice my age. Based on the choices I had for prior homecomings, I had to prepare for this great task. The task of acting like the six dresses in Dillard's was a selection, and the two in JC Penney's, left over from the holidays, was a facade. There was one inexpensive store of teen-inspired options, DEB. They had a few things, but the colors and the cuts were not right for a real plus-size girl, even if the size on the tag appeared to be plus size. The process was walking into a series of stores and walking out acting like it was just not what I wanted instead of telling the truth—there were no good choices that fit me.

The walk into each store looked something like this:

"Oh, are these the two racks you have?" I'd say.

"Yes, ma'am! Were you looking for something else?" the saleswoman would inquire.

In my mind, I would be yelling, *Hell, yeah! I need something that is* not *all black, silver, burgundy or*

ELEPHANT IN THE ROOM

sequins, below the knee, and perhaps not a full sleeve. But, I would continue the salesperson/plus-size woman dance and look at the two racks as if it were ten racks of clothes.

Then, she would lean forward, almost in a whisper, and ask, "What size are you?"

"Size twenty-two!" I'd proclaim.

"Oh, the judging *oh*, in the "someone looks at you and realizes you're a teenager, yet you wear a grown woman's size 22" tone. Well, I have these two in your size. I know they may not look good on the hanger, but I think you would like them if you tried them on."

I would try them on, still hate them, and quickly slide out of the dressing room and to the front door of the store, only to do this repeatedly. It even began to be daunting to sit in homeroom at school all the weeks before and hear girls talk about their choices and making the hard decision, but all I could think was, *At least you have a choice*. My choice was looking like the mother of the damn bride or looking like I spent thirty dollars at Rainbow, a low-priced store in the community, on a dress that I could add a shawl to make it look classy. Imagine all the size 4s complaining about the prom selection, and in my mind, I was thinking, *Hell, I can't even fit anything in the prom area!*

Imagine being sixteen years old and having to have the maturity not to hate your body, but to be rejected by every store that you entered. Prom was one of those moments that quickly taught me to expect nothing to fit just right and embrace the fact that I may have to have a more mature look than my peers. There were no junior-plus sections then to help you get a teenage look in a grown-woman body. At that time there were very few stores that had the full-figured-woman section besides department stores. So, fashion and swag had to be created, and I would have to be creative.

As the time drew near, my mom was able to identify a lady who we could order pageant dresses to size, and that's what I did! The word *pageant* is hilarious when I think of it now, but that's what they were, and I got one, and damn it, I looked good. My dress was very nice and very expensive and was a custom fit, literally! My boyfriend at the time didn't seem to mind it, and to me it was kinda sexy, in a size-22 pageant kind of way! Prom was a dress success! Even though the limo broke down so many times that we almost missed all the festivities, I had a dress that I picked, and I liked the way it fit. Prom was done, and that was the moment I knew somehow, I could get a wedding dress that would fit, too.

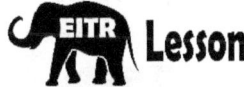 **Lesson**

Milestone moments are very different when you're plus size. Not very many people have to approach prom based on size instead of focusing on having a good time. It is not easy sitting in front of peers knowing you can't relate with their challenges with dresses because you barely had one...if they only knew your journey!

ELEPHANT IN THE ROOM

Elephant 5

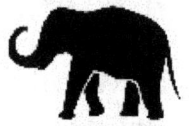

Diets!

ELEPHANT IN THE ROOM

Cabbage, Atkins, grapefruit, tuna or Jenny C! No, I'm not talking about a person or food, but these are some of the many diets in which I have participated over the years. It's funny that people think you're fat and you just refuse to do anything about it. They are so wrong! In fact, I can remember my first diet being in high school. At a time when I should be daydreaming about boys, worrying about fashion, and thinking about college, I was home dieting. My dieting plans had gotten to the point that I was on a diet all by myself and still watching my entire family continue eating as they wanted. This was when I knew my weight was *my* problem—I gained it alone, and I had to fix it alone.

I remember my aunt, my favorite aunt, who is the diet queen, sharing copies of diets with me and my dad. But the only person who was ever on a diet was me. My parents would get all the groceries I needed, and then I was on my own. I remember one time sitting down eating the grapefruit diet on a Friday night and watching my brother and parents eat a large meat lover's pizza from Pizza Hut. At that moment, I realized that the diet journey would be lonely. Everyone is together when you are eating wrong, but when it is time to sacrifice and cut calories, suddenly food is your problem.

ELEPHANT IN THE ROOM

For my fellow dieters, the road is not easy. You start off with the best intentions, all the groceries, a focused mind-set, and a plan...but somehow in the journey you feel that you don't see results, you're still hungry, and the food you have resorted to eating doesn't even taste good. Then you are back at square one, minus one less diet to have to try again. It's not that we don't want this. It's just that oftentimes it defeats us, and as anyone can tell you, it's ten times harder to get it off than it was to put it on. Even though I heard for years that eating is a lifestyle change, it has taken me sixteen years to understand I must choose better eating as a lifestyle *daily*. It is almost like acquiring all new taste buds. For me it's just trying to get through hard or stressful life moments without turning to food and making better food choices.

I want to live a food lifestyle of what Yoplait yogurt commercials call a "swapportunity." I want to take the opportunity to swap something with high calories and fried for something that is low calorie and better for me. I wanted this to come naturally. But because you grow a love affair and fondness for food that you never forget, you can lose the battle of the diet. Diets don't work, I know, but using them to begin to guide your food choices can be very helpful, and everyone needs a starting point. I would like my lifestyle to continue to evolve. I know that you have to quit looking at the diet as a long-term sacrifice but focus on each minute, hour and then the day. If I can make good choices each time, then I have changed my lifestyle for days, weeks and months. To all the diets, you have your place, but not long term with me! I must admit sometimes I want something good right now and to the gods of my waist, please be forgiving to me of my food choices. To all of you fat shamers, shame on you. You know that nothing is appeasing about a grapefruit diet to anybody, so just lay off a bit. You'll get it one day.

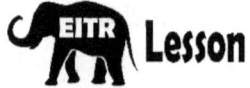 **Lesson**

I don't just sit at buffets all day, but I do like good food. Many of us have dieted for decades to fight the battle with food. We desire results, we muster all the motivation we can, but dang on it if we lose five and gain back ten. As you sometimes glare at chubby people with disdain, can you honestly admit that a carrot stick tastes better than a warm Krispy Kreme doughnut? Making that healthy choice is our struggle, and it is *real!*

Elephant 6

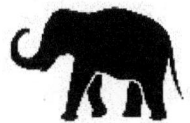

You Know Those Pants Don't Look Good on You!

ELEPHANT IN THE ROOM

I remember it was described best by Dr. Phil when the Braxton sisters were on his show, and the sisters were talking about Toni Braxton, the eldest and most famous sister. One of her issues was always having something to say. Of course, she defended herself as being the older sister and others needing the feedback, but Dr. Phil jumped right in and said, "No, it's called unsolicited feedback!" Sometimes you feel you must say something, but nobody asked you. I remember thinking, *Yes, I get that sometimes, and that is exactly what it is.* In college, I felt that same way. I received some "unsolicited feedback" and it changed my life.

I can say my that college years were the absolute best years of my life. I was finding myself and developing my voice and worldview. I was hundreds of miles away from my parents, and for once, I was not Calvin's daughter or Brandon's sister or the granddaughter of…I was just Sharita Shelby. I was lucky enough to have confidence and a strong desire to begin my marathon of life at full speed. I ran for class president. I was in honor societies. I hung with a crew called the 7SP, Seven Sister Production. I can't even remember where that name came from, but I was in the group. I was doing exactly what I set out to do when I left home. For the most part, I can say it was a smooth transition into college and a good time. I was perfectly socialized. But then a few experiences of unsolicited feedback made me think twice, and I noticed again that I was bigger than everybody else.

Let me first put out the disclaimer that *I will never give names, and I will always deny, deny, deny,* but as a college student, there are sometimes groups that you want to join. To be part of these groups, they sometimes challenge you personally, intellectually and socially. One of the groups that I wanted to be a part of "tried me," and this was all new to me. *Tried me* is a term that means something was said that was not meant for good and said to a person, me, that normally people do not challenge in that type of way and were trying to see just what my response may be. Hence, they "tried me!"

I will first start with my disclaimer. Yes, I have been heavy since the fourth grade, but no one ever talked about my weight to my face other than my family. Therefore, in that way, I had never been tried, challenged or called out. For the first time, there were outward verbal comments about me being a big girl, and I honestly had no idea how to take this. I will never forget that I ran into one of the girls already in this group I wanted to join. Because many of the

ELEPHANT IN THE ROOM

people in this group felt I was too confident, they thought they had to try to hit me where they thought it would hurt—my belly! So, I walk into a meeting held by this group, and one of the members walks up and says, "What are you doing here? Isn't there a burger special tonight at McDonald's?"

Huh? I thought as I just stood there.

First of all, I was shocked that she said it. Secondly, I was surprised she would play the weight card. Thirdly, I did have to laugh a little because the statement was clever. But in this single moment, not even thinking about my weight, since it had been on me from fourth grade, I realized it was now noticeable to her. Clearly my weight was now in range to be used as unsolicited feedback.

Was this on the minds of my classmates?

Did they think I was attending restaurants for a burger special?

Am I just a big girl to everyone?

These are the questions that flooded my mind.

I can still slightly chuckle, but this moment was real. It spoke loud and clear that as smart, funny, well adjusted, great personalitied,I know it's not a word, a

ELEPHANT IN THE ROOM

girl as I believed myself to be, people would always see my weight. As the journey in this group continued, I remember being asked to stand up. I was wearing what we called TAPs in college, which stood for tight-ass pants. These were the famous Ponte pants from Lerner of New York that came in S-XL, basically today's legging. As I stood in front of the group of my peers, a girl said, "Aren't these the pants you had on in the college fashion show?"

I said yes. Mind you, I didn't even really want to be in the college fashion show, but I pushed myself to walk the runway thinking, *Why not? What do I have to lose?* I guess I was just about to find out.

She then said, "You don't have any business wearing this type of pants. Look at how big your thighs are at the top and how small your ankle is at the bottom," as she literally used her finger to touch my thighs.

"Those pants don't look good on you!"

Well, damn! I thought everybody looked good in TAPS, but apparently not me. I will admit that it took me years to feel comfortable in a legging again. I always purchased a boot-cut Ponte pant to avoid this look that she stated I never should wear again. This one hit home more than the burger special.

ELEPHANT IN THE ROOM

For that moment, I wondered if that's how everybody saw me and, hell, how everybody saw my thighs! Here I was thinking I was a cute dresser in college, and maybe all they saw was the big thigh and the little ankle.

It's funny that I can remember this like yesterday, so in some ways this must have meant something to me and began to shape the way I felt others saw me. It was an awakening. I was not aware of what others were thinking of me and how I dressed for my size. Of course, I knew they saw me, but it never crossed my mind that I was possibly committing a lot of fashion don'ts and maybe even not representing big girls like I thought I was. I liked myself and my style, but I wasn't so sure what others saw when they looked at me. It didn't break me down in the long run. It just helped me realize I had to believe in what I put on my body, so that even if all someone else saw was a big thigh and a little ankle, I had to know and say for myself that I looked cute, nice, sexy and covered perfectly. That is how I saw myself from that day forward, but many people aren't lucky enough to pull this perspective out of this type of situation. Maybe I didn't have any business in those pants, but from that day forward, how I dressed was just that—*my business*!

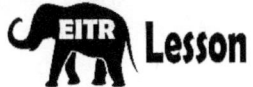 **Lesson**

As long as I like it, you better love it! I have to be comfortable in my own skin. Sometimes people can open your eyes to a perspective, but it is up to *you* to take it as the gospel of your life or leave it as just that, a *perspective!*

Elephant 7

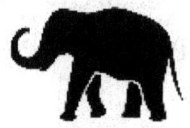

My Pull...

ELEPHANT IN THE ROOM

No arrogance included, but I have to say, I can have what I want. To all the women who look or gaze across with dismay or questions, know that for the same reason men are attracted to you, men *will be* attracted to all the *thick with-it* girls like me. Over the years, I have heard the whispers of "How? How did she get him?" But I say, maybe you should look a little harder. There is certainly more to most women than meets the eye. You see, there is nothing mysterious about it. There will always be an art to getting the attention of men, and once you understand it more deeply, being a size 6 is only one component.

The "Pull" is the ability to be noticed and sought after. This is the ability to be noticed in a group when there appears to be many other good choices.

The "Pull" is to be confident and sure of your conversation.

The "Pull" is the ability to smile and not take yourself too seriously.

The "Pull" is to be able to enjoy an evening of conversation, drinks and fun and never hint as though it matters if he asks for your number.

ELEPHANT IN THE ROOM

The "Pull" is looking nice in what you wear and walking with your head held high, knowing you have something great to offer.

Is the pull my weight? No!

The "Pull" is that I can still get all the male attention I desire, and my weight doesn't stand in the way.

With that out of the way, I want to be the first to say that at times I have said to myself, "Damn, how did I get him?"

"Oooh, what I am I going to do with him?"

Over these 37 years, I can say that even at more than 300 pounds, I still have been able to get a man. I know cheerleaders, runners, beauty queens and even some family members are hurt by my ability, but it is true! Yes, I am a big girl, but I can get me a man and sometimes your man. I do think, "Why they pick a big girl when they can have any girl?", but then I know that they are not just picking a big girl, they were choosing me! You can say what you want, but I had some "pull" in my days. They have been good-looking men, but why don't I deserve that? I do…right?

I'll never forget that I had a boyfriend in my twenties who was fine. He was bald, with beautiful caramel

ELEPHANT IN THE ROOM

skin and perfect teeth that included the most perfect gap, and he had swag! I remember bringing him to meet my family for Thanksgiving. My cousin decided to pull him to the side and take him and show him pictures of me when she felt I was not so cute and not the diva people currently described me as. She went as far as to tell him how much I had changed. She emphasized my chubby face, my Jheri curl, and just who I was in those odd preteen years.

Was she trying to embarrass me?

Get him to change his mind about being my man?

Was she trying to say that he should be with someone more like her?

Either way, this experience was the first time that I truly realized that other women had a problem with my pull. Perhaps they doubted if men were genuinely interested in me. Either way, somehow it was felt that I should have a certain type of man, and a good-looking one was not it.

I remember later one of my cousins saying to the other that he was a good-looking man and a "catch." My other cousin said, "Rita is the catch!", and in that moment, it validated me and confirmed what I always believed about myself. I was a big girl, but I was college educated at a great historically black college, funny, open minded, Christian, tall, raised in a great two-parent home, well-traveled, and my *favorite*, "well spoken", more like outspoken. So, my supportive cousin was absolutely right. I was the good catch. I may not have been a dainty goldfish, but maybe I was just a rainbow trout!

But he liked it. I liked it.

He liked me, and I liked him!

Who I am is not limited to what people see. It's much more about the spirit in me. But women, even my family, who I felt not only knew me best but were supposed to be my biggest supporters, succumbed to the world's view of what I deserved. My cousin actually took a step back and thought how a girl like me could get a man like him. Pull is so much more than size. It is the ability to use words right, the art of laughter, and the depth of my soul that people are intrigued about ... and of course my thickness! I will not act like I'm not good-looking. I have great height, nice lips, okay skin, and I ... am ... attractive. So, why not me? *I got pull!*

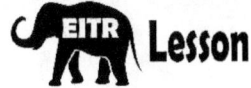 **Lesson**

Be confident in who you are! The outside doesn't determine your worth, *and* there are many men who like a woman with hips, thighs and plenty of butt. The more *you* demonstrate that *you* like who you are, the more they like you!

You got *pull!*

Elephant 8

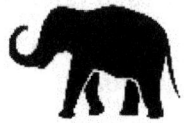

Biggirlswithgoodcredit.com

ELEPHANT IN THE ROOM

There was an advertisement on a famous syndicated radio show that advertised for big girls with good credit. The ad included a checklist about getting a fat girl to finance your desires. For example:

You can't get a car financed? Call a big girl.

You wanna go out to eat at a five-star restaurant for free? Call a big girl.

You need a house, or an apartment approved? Call a big girl.

Basically, they're saying you could use a big girl. Even though there may have been a chuckle the very first time I heard it, I thought it was a real ad on the radio and was completely caught off guard. The thought of it is extremely interesting and damn near degrading. It was saying if a man lowered his physical-attribute standards, he could be on a "come up" with a fat woman. The ad encouraged men who like thick girls to find a big girl, who would have low self-esteem, and use her for his financial gain. This was an advertisement to tell you how to get over on someone else? What the hell!

ELEPHANT IN THE ROOM

This bothered me because:

You would never hear an ad about somebody who was extremely skinny with no butt and a child-size chest.

You would never hear an ad about someone facially unfortunate, a.k.a. ugly.

You most *certainly* would not hear an ad about anyone with a disability or an "outwardly noticeable disability."

Yet, it was okay to exploit and joke about someone who is overweight? This ad saw big women as low-self-esteemed fat girls who would consider it an honor and a privilege to be taken advantage of because their clothes tag said XXL, giving life to believing that we have money saved to be used for others as our way of securing our men? Please.

After hearing this ad, I had a conversation with someone about it. She gave the look like, "Yeah, that is why some men choose big girls—just to use them!" The more I started to think about what she said, considering she was a slightly thick woman herself, led me to be further disappointed in our fellow women. Did the thought of preference ever cross anyone's mind in the area of looks? Some men like

ELEPHANT IN THE ROOM

tall, short, boobs, butt, teeth, eyes, light skin, chocolate skin—so why wouldn't they like someone heavier? Why didn't the possibility ever cross anyone's mind that maybe he is a man that loves a pretty face. Therefore, he doesn't focus so much on the body, or maybe he likes something to grab onto during sex or a soft body lying next to him. A man does not have to resort to a plus-size woman, so he can use her. Just maybe that is what he likes and exactly what he wants! I also was disappointed that she was saying it was a given and synonymous to being used. Being used has more to do with self-concept and boundaries than it has to do with any physical attributes. If you are the kind of woman that allows men to use you, then that is just who you are. If men need a "come up" and they seek out someone to assist them because they are not willing to do it, then it is more than settling for fat. It is an extreme character flaw on their part. You can go to the website fatgirlswithgoodcredit.com, but you just might be redirected to brokemenwhocan'ttakecareofthemselves.org.

So, let me clear this up once and for all:

First, many men do what we call "frontin'," which is slang for stating something in the presence of others to make them believe a certain thing about you, and

ELEPHANT IN THE ROOM

most of the time it is not true. There are many, *many* men that like thick girls and who have certainly liked me. And, they are not just the heavy boys or the painfully shy guys from your science class or the facially challenged men. These are *your* men! The ones that are fine, are educated, have great conversation, are independent, go to church, are artistically talented, and even your gym rats. This frontin' has allowed men and too many women to believe that big girls are third-choice citizens when we are not! If a man wants to pursue you, then *he will*. Your size will have nothing to do with it, and on the low, it may have everything to do with it.

Skinny readers, can you say that you haven't been used, or that because of your weight you have had a better pool of men? Um, not really, I just know it. I do realize that in a conversation with others it would be more befitting of a man to dote on Halle Berry versus Monique, but secretly you like what you like and love who you love. Men don't front. And, ladies, please do not allow your personal insecurities to cause you to talk down plus-sized women, especially when half of you will be one someday!

ELEPHANT IN THE ROOM

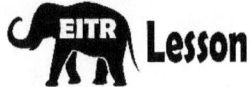 **Lesson**

It's not my credit they chose, it's *me*. It's not my weight that defines his attraction, it's *me*. It's not settling for *me*, it's liking *me*. Men choose all kinds of women, and they choose *me*!

ELEPHANT IN THE ROOM

Elephant 9

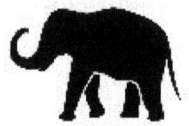

What Was That?

ELEPHANT IN THE ROOM

Okay, okay, okay, this chapter is dedicated to the exact moment when you have gone too far and are not sure how to come back. The moment you sit in a chair, stand on something, try to pull on some article of clothing and you hear a noise indicating something has snapped, cracked, torn or broken. This can be the most embarrassing moment, but your mere hope is that you are the only one who has heard it or seen it.

This moment is normally brought to you by the plastic chairs that are at the family barbeque or the tag in that shirt at the mall that is misrepresenting what you feel is your size. When you sit down in the chair, your first hope is that it can hold you and the legs don't bend. Once you master that, you pray that things are good from that moment on—then you hear a crack! For the most part, nothing changes. You are still seated, but you know somewhere something has been damaged. You are praying that it's only something you heard and not something you will have to see or experience.

All furniture is a test of durability, from your bed frame to your dining-room chairs. I even found myself looking over people's furniture subconsciously to decide where my butt was going to have the best fit. When you walk into a place with cheap furniture, you immediately hope this is not the

ELEPHANT IN THE ROOM

beginning of a tragic incident. This moment also happens with clothes in a dressing room. There have been times that outside of damn near breaking into a sweat to get something pulled on, there has been the sound of a split, tear, and even an airborne button. Now to stick up for myself here, yes, I know my size. However, when you know the market of plus-size shopping, you learn very quickly that every size 22 is not created equal. You slide, or should I say, attempt to slide your butt in the size 20 that you really want to be because it's cute, and doggone it, you want it! This dressing-room escapade is silently embarrassing, and then there is the moment where you get upset with yourself.

Why, when it first felt tight, did I not stop trying to pull on this outfit?

After you get this experience planted in your subconscious, you learn the art of trying things that look possibly too tight on so that you don't bust a zipper or loosen a seam. I know when to pull something over my head, step in or wiggle it down.

There are a few articles of clothing that I put on that almost make me want to cry to get out of because for some reason, even when I try to bend my arm, I can't get out. When you finally get it over your head, your

ELEPHANT IN THE ROOM

face is warm to due to the squeeze trying to get it over your head, and your hair looks like you just woke up from a deep sleep. Usually, you need to exhale. On both ends of the noises -the tear in the clothes or my groaning- and tears, I'm just someone who wants to try something on, but the devil of weight just wants to take me out of my shopping happy place. Next thing I know, I am looking around the dressing room, praying that no one has seen or heard it. And praying that the lady in the next room isn't yelling out, "What was that?"

Can you imagine your life of trying on clothes or going places only to have to keep the thought of *Will I break or damage anything?* As these scenarios roll out of my mind and on this paper, I realize it is my normal.

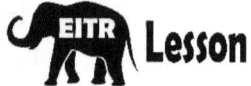 **Lesson**

Being a big girl is a lifestyle. You not only have to navigate the world of clothes but the world of furniture! Something must be able to hold you and support you and by all means never break or embarrass you. Ladies, may the force be with you as you navigate this. And, to our friends, the hosts of events, give us a break. We don't want to break the furniture.

Elephant 10

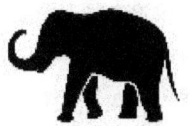

Black Girls Don't Run!

ELEPHANT IN THE ROOM

Of course, we don't run! Our hair can't handle those types of conditions! No, but seriously, I was at work one day in a company where all of us were known for having conversations that were too honest. During one of those work conversations, one of the guys said, "You know what the problem with black women is? They don't exercise or take care of themselves, and they don't care about letting their bodies go!"

Well, of course that did not sit well with me. I began to speak about the preferences of my thickness to all the men that loved my softness and curves, and then my thoughts grew deeper about what had been said. Was it true that we didn't care about our bodies and that was why we were larger than many of our Caucasian counterparts? Hell no! Our weight isn't that simple. I can give three reasons why it seems as if we may not look like our counterparts or seem to take the same level of interest!

1. **We did not grow up with the food education on healthy eating.** We grew up with Granny and Big Momma, who knew the art of soul-food cooking and the blessed skills to make a cake that was the best you ever had. The love in our families was not always demonstrated through the hugs and kisses and affirmative

words all the time but through the time, energy, effort and care that it took to cook these great dishes. This was generational learning. No one was teaching Big Momma about low carbs, the food triangle, or the importance of working out. Our grandparents were born in a time where there wasn't always enough food and often did not have the choices of the most nutritious food, so they doctored up, seasoned well, what they had. Do you think there is any other reason that we could love chitlins ,chitterlings—pig intestines? Uh, no!

2. **Due to the demanding life that many lived, being raised by a single parent or getting the education, time and commitment that it took to be independently successful, our parents redirected their focus to surviving and not nutritionally thriving.** Our parents were first-generation college attendees. They were trying to find the glass ceiling and figure out how to at least get into the building, while their counterparts' husbands were getting good jobs and already living sustainable lifestyles. Our counterparts' parents also paid for them to attend college, receive internships,

and land careers through their business associates. The women were also taught to marry into families who could afford them a stay-at-home lifestyle. When you're not afforded the opportunity of a stay-at-home lifestyle, running on a treadmill is not at the top of your priority list. But being a first-generation success is!

3. **We were raised to love our curves!** Unlike many of our counterparts, we are proud to have thick thighs and voluptuous butts and breasts. All the jokes in our culture shun those of us who are rail thin and flat chested with no butts. So why work to get rid of this physique? Yes, as women we all think we can stand to lose a few pounds, but for us, curves are beautiful and have defined us since the beginning of time.

When the guys said that we are uninterested in our bodies, they were wrong. We are! And finally, we have a generation of women who have carved out time in the gym, learning what clean eating even is and working to implant health awareness and fitness into our kids. On the other hand, the numbers don't lie, and yes, black women may carry a few more pounds, but also there are record numbers of women

ELEPHANT IN THE ROOM

all over the world getting two of the most common enhancement surgeries: breast augmentation and butt implants. So, guys, maybe you are slightly hypocritical when you say you want us to work out more, but you certainly are asking for bigger boobs and bigger butts!

One of the movements that has taken off is Black Girls Run, and I like it because it is a declaration toward black women that our health and our bodies are important to us. It is slightly frustrating to know that we have to claim this declaration for people to believe that we have a desire to be healthy and fit. So, I will say that yes, I am more of a Zumba girl than a runner, but yes, black girls do run … just not me!

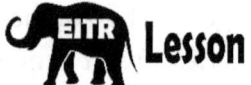 **Lesson**

Before you speak, just think for a minute. Things aren't always as simple as they appear. Weight and healthy living was not always at the forefront of our journey, but that doesn't make us less than our counterparts or uninterested. It just makes us constant evolvers. Black girls rock, and now they run. So, now what's the problem?

ELEPHANT IN THE ROOM

Elephant 11

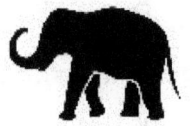

Spandex, All Spandex

ELEPHANT IN THE ROOM

Yes, Lord! I am talking about a girdle! SPANX! Good old-fashioned undergarments! Who needs them? You, me, us! One thing I can say is, even with my full-figured body, I have made sure that there are no lumps, bumps or clumps. And this was all due to the Spandex god. Just enough Lycra to hold me in and just loose enough to breathe once every thirty minutes. If you have not found yourself a girdle, then you and your clothes are missing out.

I remember when I was in college and I was putting on the Big G, and one of my friends said, "Of course I don't have a girdle; my stomach is not big like that." That statement stopped me dead in my tracks. Even my mother, who was a size 8, put on a girdle, and this friend of mine was a couple of sizes bigger than that.

So, it caused me to ponder, *at what size should a woman wear a girdle?*

Well, after much pondering and praying, I'm going to go with an 8. After this point, something is starting to grow outside of the regular proportions. Am I saying you are overweight at a size 8? Absolutely not! But can your clothes and body use a little squeeze to make your clothes fit well and look

ELEPHANT IN THE ROOM

smooth on you? Yes! Lately, I have seen more dimpled butts, thighs and post baby stomachs than I ever wanted to see. You certainly have an excuse for the weight—you brought a beautiful baby in this world, or your love of great food caused your body to stretch in unexpected ways. However, either way, it is time for the Big G.

My girlfriend had a good shape, but in her dresses, I could always see her belly hanging out, and deep inside I wanted her to join me. I could even see the belly-button cut out. Does she not see what I see? I guess what plagues me is, what is the reflection that many see in the mirror? Even when I slid into a size 28, it was a lot of woman in my clothes, but it was a smooth woman. I think people may say "It's just my stomach. Besides that, I'm good." Well, what I want to say is, the stomach is where obesity rears its ugly head 75 percent of the time. There are only thighs and arms left to qualify.

By no means am I suggesting all our stomachs be flat, but I am suggesting letting all our thickness be smooth. I am my mother's child, and many women did not have the luxury of growing up with a woman who always wore pantyhose with a skirt and a girdle, who was smaller than most people. Lycra to my mother was a part of good lady decorum. Any

ELEPHANT IN THE ROOM

woman should want her clothes to just fall on her instead of cushion and fit every roll and dimple to size. Women will be in the cutest, short, booty-showing, cleavage-enhancing dress but will leave out the most important element: *spandex!*

Ladies, we need spandex. She is our friend, and even she must fit. Girdles come in sizes too, and there is no need to try to fool yourself with your smoothing garment. I have seen a few people attempting the Big G but didn't get the one best for their body. It looked like they had two or three stomachs instead of one that the girdle covers. I can admit it. I have at least seven girdles, all specializing in different areas. I have a panty girdle and a high-waist panty girdle. I have girdle boy shorts and girdle capris. I have one that goes all the way to my boobs, for that fat roll right under my breasts. Then, I have two that I literally break out in a sweat when I put them on. I have to pull those out when I'm really in need of some assistance.

Ladies, don't be afraid to be smooth, and don't let the cost of a girdle deter you. Girdles are our friends. They don't say we're fat. They simply say we like to look smooth. The Big Gs are in your local Walmart and most stores with a lingerie section. They are in most plus-size lingerie/underwear stores since you smaller ladies aren't exactly grabbing them off the shelves.

Mirdle

I just couldn't resist speaking briefly about the man girdle. Ladies, this is the best example of simply desiring to be smooth, I guess. Men would never admit it out loud, but some of them have a little boobage and more belly than they need, and secretly they are wearing a "mirdle." I must admit that one of my man friends had one. We never talked about it, and to be honest I thought it was a traditional tank top undershirt, culturally known as a wife beater, I know it is a totally inappropriate title, but hey, I didn't create it. I noticed, in an effort to get it off of him, one day I felt some of that old-fashioned spandex and knew it was a "mirdle." He honestly was not the heaviest guy I dated and was one of the most confident ones, but I was exposed to his little man secret. I don't know how many men are wearing these and singing, *"It ain't nothing but a G thing, baby!"*

I know this is the extreme opposite of what Dr. Dre and Snoop Dogg had in mind. I am all for the mirdles, but it does tell me just how much image does not just live with the ladies anymore. In fact, thoughts of weight and imperfect perfections are creeping in men's heads, too. The very people that we work so hard to impress and be perfect for suddenly feel inadequate about their bodies and are willing to buy a mirdle just for the appearance of being smoother. I must say there are few more men that may need to slide into their first mirdle. Smooth, baby, I want it all smooth!

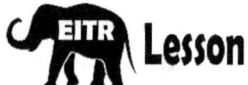 **Lesson**

Be comfortable in the skin you're in, but roll it out and keep it smooth. Nothing can deceive the eye of weight more than smoothing it out for your outfit. It can be uncomfortable and doggone restrictive, but the product is awesome! The product is you, and even though people look at our weight, it sure it helps when we represent it well by wearing our clothes and not always allowing the clothes to wear us.

ELEPHANT IN THE ROOM

Elephant 12

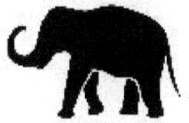

These Ain't Your Mama's Rolls

ELEPHANT IN THE ROOM

They just keep moving! No matter what you to do tame them, it's hard to keep them contained. When you think you've got one, another one forms, and you begin to make body parts that have never existed before. You can try Lycra, spandex, firm cotton or just double up on clothing, but whatever you do, you must cover them up. What are these things I speak of?

Rolls! Not your mama's rolls that are accompanied with gravy or grape jam, but those places where all the bad food you've eaten or even thought about eating live.

I have to admit, they drive me crazy! You already know how I feel about girdles. Every woman who walks the earth should have at least one. But the culprit is not spandex, it's those damn rolls. They are on your sides, the bottom of your back, even one under your breasts. Is it not enough, Lord, just to be fat and have to squeeze a body in a jean where the tag reads size 28? But then, to go manage to look smooth as you temper your fat is a challenge within itself. Because rolls hold relatively soft tissue, they can get away from you. If you put on a stomach girdle, you can be left with a back roll. If you try just a panty girdle, an extra stomach can form. And even if you put on a full-body girdle, these things will roll

ELEPHANT IN THE ROOM

out from up under your arms. I like a roll, it rises and works best with jam. But, jamming these rolls right into place ... that's some work! I have a girdle that goes to your knees, but you can even create a roll around your knees.

How unnatural is that?

I mean seriously, how do you get a knee roll?

When you try to tame big thighs and the girdle is just a little tight, it forms. Now, if you are skinny, I imagine you may not know about this, but trust me when I say this shit is unbelievable. One time I had to wear a long-line bra and full, step-in girdle to wear a cute red dress I purchased. There was a small space in between the two, and what do you know — a new roll appears. I preach Lycra, but it is more than a notion to control the rolls. These plague us sassy voluptuous women who just wanna look good in our clothes, but then there is another feature on the body menu that comes next: the skin and the double chin.

My dad always says, he is like my personal Martin Luther King Jr., "If you have a small face or head, people don't think you are as fat, no matter how big your body is." Those of us with that fat face are already put in the fat-people category. This is a little perplexing but a truth of a chubby-faced, fat person.

ELEPHANT IN THE ROOM

We have all seen those women with the short haircut, chiseled chin, dimples, thin lips, and the cutest little face, only to be stunned when you look six inches down and see a triple-D chest and the ankles that fall over their size-6 foot. I love all thick women, but that small face is a small pass to people thinking you aren't that big, even if you kind've are.

Even among the heavy community, there is still discrimination against each other. There are different kinds of thickness. The huge-chested woman, the all-stomach-silhouette woman, the fat-face-with-the-triple-chin woman, the under-five-foot heavy woman, the six-foot-plus-with-the-size-12-feet woman, the small-waist-but-huge-butt woman, and the box-shape-with-no-true-waist woman. I could name a few more, but you get the picture. In each of these categories, you must figure out how to put your best hips, waist, chest and foot forward. When you know you have a double chin, you have to go in double-chin-reduction training. How this works is in the mirror you practice smiles and a look that doesn't cause your double chin to hang as low. At least, I did. In the day of selfies, usies, and unknown video footage, you must sit on ready when it comes to photographic documentation. You may need to look up more, straighten your back so your neck will

ELEPHANT IN THE ROOM

elongate, and sometimes learn the right face slant to make it appear less fat. This is serious business in the age of selfies.

But we can't stop there.

There are also ways to hide all the excess skin from those flabby arms and those thunder thighs. The game changer was the girdle/Spanx and the sleeve lol. One of my friends has even gotten the science down of holding the arm flab of the person in front of you in group photos to reduce the arm-fat shot. This always has me laughing, but it works. The thing is, when there is a lot of dough in the cake, fat on our bodies, the skin has to have somewhere to go, so it stretches, folds, dimples and creates rolls. As a plus-size woman in America, or any other woman, we must acquire the art of adjusting our bodies for just the right look in the new world of documentation also known as social media. In a world where hiding is no longer an option, you just have to get ready. So, if you have the chin and skin, like me, maybe there should be classes to learn how to alter our appearance of these love muffins on our bodies, or maybe we can just stick with the few pointers listed above. No matter what we can strut, strut, strut, and we just do our best to give the best look we got, even if it's a grin and a double chin.

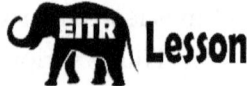 **Lesson**

Stand up straight, slight head tilt, hands on your hips or as close to you as possible, and always suck in your stomach. This is the work for the perfect picture. But the true picture is the smile and the feelings you convey on your photos. I know it feels like the new life checklist, but of course it omits one thing, the confidence of the model! You are the model so just give it your best and what you really got, beyond that roll, will shine through.

ELEPHANT IN THE ROOM

Elephant 13

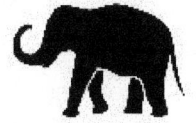

Out to Eat

ELEPHANT IN THE ROOM

It is America's favorite pastime. It is the place where birthdays are celebrated, where girls' nights are built, and the place where moms across the world get to just sit and enjoy the culinary efforts of others. It is going out to eat! It is something that we do all day, every day. But there is a challenge to this activity of daily living. Despite all of the advertisements for indulgences of great food, we hear very little about the restaurant and its amenities. We have the largest portion sizes in the world but sometimes the smallest, most uncomfortable seats. There is something not right with that picture, and it's more than the size of my ass. All the preparation to eat at my favorite restaurant and now I gotta sit down and think about how I can get into their seats? It all begins with a trip to your local eatery and they ask your name, and then the challenge begins.

"Would you like a table or a booth?"

This is the big question ... that your butt, hips, and thighs are waiting for you to answer just to see how comfortable they will be.

A booth, well, that is typically the most comfortable, but if the table is built connected to the bench, you can be so close to the table that you can barely breathe. The table with chairs, well that's typically a good choice unless you are at one of the savvy, swank restaurants that have an armrest that squeezes you in or the chair is damn near plastic and you're praying that it doesn't crack, squeak or move before you get good and seated. The split-second decision could literally weigh on how I feel the next day by being bruised from the squeezing of the armrest or my butt hurts from sitting in the chair. This immediately brings up the thought of one of my favorite places to eat.

There is no place on earth that we all love to go to more than the Cheesecake Factory! Known for an elaborate menu, large portions and even an Oreo cheesecake! But on many occasions, I had to sit in their plastic wicker-style chairs that always leave a bruise on my outer thighs because of this tight chair. But who could turn down this restaurant? And when you are with women who are equally as fluffy, someone must sit in those chairs, even if one side gets the bench seating. To eat at this place, I also must choose to have bruises and soreness the next day.

I am sure when the designers of these restaurants think of what is sleek and fits with the ambience that they want to create, the last thing on their mind is to select chairs for all sizes. It is nowhere on their radar that the people that love to eat might have a little

ELEPHANT IN THE ROOM

more junk in the trunk and will need a great place to sit all of it. They are not the only culprits. Some of these new modern-day barstools without the backs are bad too. Not only do they cause you to slide all over the seat but then you must make sure your ass is not hanging off of it. And if you have big boobs, which I don't have to worry about, they can practically be laid out on the table like an appetizer, depending on the height of the table. Most people go right in to these great restaurants without any anxiety, but if you are on the heavy side, you already know the possible obstacle that can be presented. For those of you who go out to eat with us, maybe you can just look around before you select where we sit. When you are out the next time with someone that has a little more size, choose wisely, just go with a table and look at the chair style, so that they don't lose the fight with the battle of the ill-fitting chair!

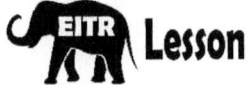 **Lesson**

If you never walked a day in my shoes or, for that matter, sat a day in my seat, you will never know my struggle. Something never thought about by the average American can be a barrier to enjoying the most social place in America, the dining table. Sometimes people may not be choosing not to hang out with you. They just may be choosing to not be uncomfortable in that chair at your favorite restaurant all night.

Elephant 14

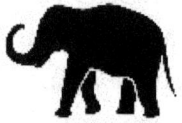

What's Been Eating Her?

ELEPHANT IN THE ROOM

I hate to say it but … I've been plus sized my whole life. In some ways it is very much a part of who I am. For those of you who grew into this, I will give you my condolences. I can't imagine being a size six or ten in high school and looking at a 22/24 tag later in life. It must be overwhelming and slightly embarrassing. Do know that your size is not who you are, but it does begin to be part of our story. I am sure that you are experiencing life a little differently now that you are on the other side of the scale … I mean the store … I mean life. You probably never knew your legs could stay rubbing together or that your belly could rest on your coo. It's downright depressing. But please, please, once you join us, don't spend all your time talking about still being a six. It drives me crazy. I have sat through countless conversations listening to women brag about what size they used to be. Is it because they think I will secretly be envious that they weren't always in the big girls' club? Or do they not want to renounce their membership in the skinny club? Well, all I do is look at you with concern, hoping you can handle this life. I look to see how much strength you have in you because it's not easy having the world stare, glare and compare because you're heavy.

ELEPHANT IN THE ROOM

I know you wonder how this happened and why someone didn't do or say something. Well, you see, weight is one of those things that no one speaks about until you have gotten too big. Yes, people notice, but is it really a friend's place to say, "Girl, you've gained weight!" They think you see it too, so there's no need to bring it up, right?

I hate to admit I have commented on people who have gained a lot a weight with the disclaimer, "Well, I know I'm big, but I've been big all my life, so I know ain't nobody gonna say shit to me."

And to some extent, I am right! The only people who had the heart to address me were my parents, and they normally started with health. My dad would just flat out say, "Oooh, you really would be fine if you lost 50 pounds!"

My mom would just ask, "Have you been to the gym lately?", or "Do you like salads?"

I'm laughing to myself as I type because there aren't a lot of kind ways to truly address this. Yes, this was a little challenging for me to hear, but they are the only ones who would say it. They were the mirror to my obesity. But it is more than what was said. It was my time to start thinking through what I wanted to do.

ELEPHANT IN THE ROOM

As you look at the new you, I know it is hard to see that young, chiseled face and chin you used to have, or to be speechless at the thought of your favorite high-school jeans that you now can't even dream about putting a leg in. Now you have to muster up the courage to know that things have changed but you are still you. There is grief involved with weight gain because you were once small and never even thought about weight or size. You are grieving a lifestyle that you once had. You look at yourself with slight shame and wonder how things got this bad. It takes time to grieve and more time to be angry, rationalize and finally accept this foreign body, but you will. Remember that your weight is just a suit, but you can change your wardrobe. It is ten times harder to lose weight than it ever was to gain it. But the journey to acceptance and change gives you back ten times more confidence to know you stood up to your body changing and either chose to embrace the new you or chose to change things for yourself. Either way, the lesson is in the acceptance. So, don't worry about *what* has been eating you, but instead think of how you will not allow what you eat to define who you are. Food serves as an invisible relationship in our life. Due to its content, the result of a poor relationship with food results physically on our bodies. So, explore your relationship and how it can be redefined to exhibit what you want in your life.

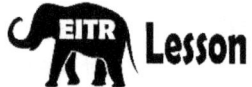 **Lesson**

Boy, do things change. I have never even had the luxury of being a size 6, so feel blessed if you have. But I'm sure to even have to learn of Lane Bryant can be hard on your psyche. Know that size does not define you, but confidence does. So the day you wake up and don't feel confident, work to change what you don't like. Don't let the shame eat you.

Elephant 15

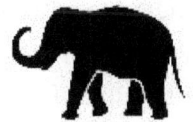

Seat-Belt Extender

ELEPHANT IN THE ROOM

Traveling is my favorite thing to do. I love the thought of leaving my life a few times a year to venture to a new place that I have never been and a part of the world that I have never experienced and most important has never experienced me. I begin each trip with a down-to-the-hour itinerary of what I want to accomplish, and then I purchase outfits appropriate for each leg of my trip. To most, that may already be mentally exhausting, but it's exciting and exhilarating for me, and it never gets old. But, before I get to my destination, I have to *fly*, and for a heavy woman, that can be a task within in itself. Luckily for me I have height, so it reduces my width, my overall appearance of width, at least. However, when it's time to get on a plane, there certainly cannot be people with too much width sitting side by side, or it is definitely going to be a very up-close and personal flight. Not only am I praying that I am not sitting next to another weight-challenged person, but I'm also hoping everything will go well with the seat belt. On some planes, I can juuust get the seat belt fastened, but on others I am an inch or two too big, and that means, the journey of getting a seat-belt extender now begins.

First let me say as soon as fat people get on the plane, everyone on the plane is praying and even enduring

ELEPHANT IN THE ROOM

a middle seat so that they don't sit by the "big one." As you do the walk of shame down the plane aisle, everyone is looking you up and down from head to toe with that short smile and asking God to let this person *not* have to sit next to them, just like, I guess, the same prayer I am praying about the woman with the baby.

As you walk on, you're immediately trying to find the flight attendant so that you can make eye contact with them so that you can ask for the seat extender without having to yell it out. But of course, it is a tropical-looking woman who is a size 6 and has selective hearing, which requires that you speak louder so that you can be completely embarrassed. Not only do you have to get past the asking point, but often the seat extenders are all the way in the front of the plane. Now the tropical flight attendant walks past 27 rows to reach over two people you're sitting with to hand you the seat-belt extender, and at that point you just wish you were invisible.

As many times as I wished I was invisible, nothing embarrasses me more because now the whole plane has verified that I'm overweight and can't even get the seat belt to fit. Then I just smile and clip it on as if it is not a big deal because normally I'm flying alone and don't know anyone on the plane. But for goodness sake couldn't this flight attendant spare me the humiliation of holding it above the seat so everyone can see for 27 rows!

Here you are sitting in a situation where you are different from everyone around you, and at a single moment, everyone will know it. Everyone has their insecurities, but on a plane, there is only one thing that you cannot hide, and that is your size and that this aircraft seat was not made for you. Now everyone on the plane knows it. The seat-belt extender is symbolic of "you just don't fit." And when you don't fit, you know it, and it is not helpful for others to feel the need to point it out. There are thousands of people smaller than me who refuse to fly because they have to face this just to go on a vacation.

One day I had a thought.

Could I just buy my own seat-belt extender?

Actually, I would love it in pink! Therefore, I wouldn't have to deal with the mood of a flight attendant. And to all those people who let out the sighs, you need to just mind your own damn business. Just because it appears that I love good food does not mean that I should have to stay at home and not get on a plane.

One of my favorite Tyler Perry movies, *Why Did I Get Married?*, illustrates this as the character drives hundreds of miles to her destination alone just because she could not "fit into her seat" and there was no availability for her to purchase two plane tickets to accommodate her size. This was not only humiliating for her, but it even shed light on the situation with her weight and her husband. We all know that your spouse/companion is aware of your weight and has made "little suggestions" about how you need to work on it. But now, even when traveling, these moments just highlight it for you, *and* for them that they were right, and now one hundred plane passengers are there to give their eye confirmation. Yes, eye confirmation is when there are no words said, but the eye of judgement and disappointment cover you when people look at your size and this situation. As much as I can understand why sitting next to the big person for two hours may feel uncomfortable, it's just as bad for me to sit next to the lady that won't stop talking, the man that accidently lays on my shoulder, or getting hit with the damn drink cart because I am near six feet tall and the flight attendant can't seem to steer it straight.

ELEPHANT IN THE ROOM

Thank you to the few flight attendants who have discreetly gotten the extender to my seat and have

given me the underhand pass. Life is inconvenient for many of us, but for this two hours in your life, just be inconvenienced.

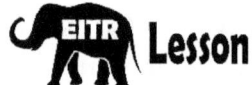 **Lesson**

Life is inconvenient for many of us, especially when traveling. But you decide what role you will play the next time you give eye confirmation when it comes to humiliating others as it pertains to their size. Remember, they already feel worse than you, so the sighs, stares and glares really don't help. And don't forget weight has a sneaky way of coming on all of us, and one day it could be you requesting the infamous seat extender!

Elephant 16

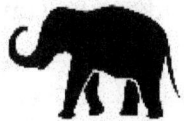

The Size of Adventure

ELEPHANT IN THE ROOM

I love to travel. What can I say? My plan is to make it to all fifty states before I die, and let's say I've been to more than half. It is something about getting on a plane and going someplace where you have never been, doing something you have never done, with people who have no idea who you are. I don't know why this excites me so much, but the thought of it almost makes my heart skip a beat. I guess because most of my life, I have "followed the rules," and I am a creature of habit and an "extreme planner," so getting away is my time to tap into the unfollowed rules of my soul—but of course with an itinerary. Stateside travel is great, but I can also say that I have finally even begun to get a few stamps on my passport, too.

As you travel abroad, you get introduced to world excursions. Excursions are mini-adventures that you pay additional cost for at any resort. These are often the defining moments of your trip, unless you are the type of person that goes on vacation to eat, sleep and drink. Maybe that's what I've been missing all these years, relaxing! Excursions include anything from swimming with dolphins, horseback riding, riding ATVs and zip-lining. These adventures range from about seventy-five dollars a person to about three hundred dollars per person, but they look like so much fun and are damn worth it. As you arrive to your hotel, you are normally greeted by the "resort concierge," and they send a representative to meet with you to schedule an excursion. As you peruse through the brochures, you are sure to find an adventure that you saw on television and now are suddenly granted this premier opportunity to participate.

Now, that I have traveled a few places, I look forward to what adventure will be hosted in the new place I visit. Being the planner I am, I usually check online to the see the high-level offerings, but I wait for the infamous brochure to make my decision. I finally meet with the vacation representative and sit at the table with my cash in hand, and now I'm ready.

"I think I would like to do the horseback-riding excursion including the forest scenery and the beach tour. I would like to take the morning trip, please," I say with confidence.

"Yes, ma'am! You have made an excellent choice, but I do have to advise you of something. In order to participate in the horse excursion, there is a weight limit 250 pounds. I am not suggesting this is your weight, but I am required to tell you this."

"Wow! Okay, well, I guess I can do something else. Can I see the brochures again?"

In that moment, I felt like I weighed one ton because not only was I slightly embarrassed, but I also felt that suddenly I would not have the opportunity to have my dream vacation.

"Well, is that drop-dead weight, or is that just the number they give you?" I ask.

"Ma'am, I'm not sure, but they ask us *not* to send people if we think they are over the maximum weight."

Suddenly, I shrink again, but I just respond. "Oh, that's okay. I understand."

I mean, I do understand that horses are animals and I am sure that there is only so much weight that they can handle to move, but I guess I just never thought the limit would be me. I wish that I could say that this was just one isolated excursion, at one resort, but it wasn't. As I have become more traveled, I have learned which things aren't designed for heavy girls. Zip-lining, horseback riding and even ATVs have a weight limit. So, you mean my weight matters everywhere, even in paradise? Who knew there was even a size for adventure.

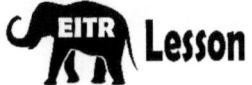 **Lesson**

Even in whimsical paradise, where I am supposed to leave all my cares behind for just a moment, I am reminded again that I'm not like everybody else. Next time I'll try a beach massage, snorkeling or a museum tour. I may just have to redefine my adventure to fit me.

Elephant 17

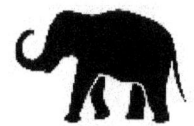

Three Hundred and You're Done!

ELEPHANT IN THE ROOM

Okay, my hope is that there are some people who don't even know that 300 pounds is the highest number on most scales, even in the doctor's office. Who knew that I would ever have to worry about that, but, shamefully I have to say I have been there.

I can remember being in my physician's office and being 298 pounds, thinking to myself, *Oh, shit. What is going to happen next?* Since I can have a dramatic mind at times, all I could think about was the scale that they use on all the obesity shows, when they must take the 500-pound person to the post office or some warehouse to weigh them. I thought that an extra Zumba class or one less cookie could keep me off the scale of shame. I hoped this would finally motivate me for the long run and I would do it. I would finally lose weight so that I would never get to 300.

Well, I attempted that, but unfortunately there came the day that I was 300 pounds, and to my surprise I didn't have to go to the post office. My doctor had these small weights that she would add in increments of ten for anyone more than 300 pounds. The nurse did not even comment once I jumped over the three-hundred-pound mark. She just reached over and added the weights. Even though she looked over it so quickly, I didn't, and I couldn't help but to think, *How did I get here?* Inside this was a moment of shame, and even though no one else knew, I knew. What would I say at the DMV, or when I had to fill out the insurance sheet? This was the infamous weight where officially I couldn't just say I was heavy. I felt obese. The scale experience may have begun in the doctor's office, but moving forward I couldn't go anywhere to get weighed because now I was over 300 pounds, and most scales only go to 300 and some even less than that. I have even gotten on a scale when it was like the scale refused to answer. It was digital, so it just started flashing what looked like all zeros. Now most of us 300 pounders may not be the ones out shopping for scales, but it is another big-girl challenge that is hard to overlook. This does something to the inside of you. I feel that I am a confident woman, but in these moments, it is overwhelming to process the contradiction between your self-acceptance and this scale that yells, "Houston we have a problem!"

No matter how well you dress your weight or how socially accepted you may be, the scale places a whole new challenge on your life. It is walking around knowing there is a discrepancy between the two. Yes, yes, yes, you know that you need to change something, but you just aren't quite sure how to help yourself. Your relationship with food has now betrayed you because it no longer just tastes good. It has begun to shape your life experiences. There are limits to where you can go and what you can do. I appreciate the reality check of the scale, but I can also say it is a sure downer of your esteem. The one thing I hate is limits, and as these things begin to get forced on me, I knew that I would have to make a change to gain my freedom and power back one day.

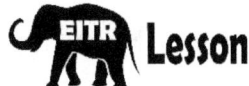 **Lesson**

It's not easy when you see a number on a scale. You know that number defines you for others, but it also has a way of confining areas of your self-confidence. The day that number changes you on the inside, then consider what adjustments you want to make on the outside.

ELEPHANT IN THE ROOM

Elephant 18

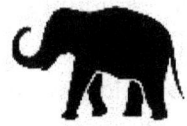

Hypochondriac

ELEPHANT IN THE ROOM

Shortness of breath? Check!

Difficulty breathing? Check!

Difficulty sleeping? Check!

Pain in my big left toe? Check!

This was me when I would go through the symptoms, you know, like part of every commercial for any new diagnosis or pain medication. I would be self-diagnosed in 120 seconds. Now, with technology I have been given WebMD, and for me that was just as good as attending John Hopkins University and getting my medical degree. Everything I even think I have is explained with cause, symptoms, treatment and of course how to pronounce it to others so that I can be sure when I inform my doctor and my friends of my ailments.

I have been to the emergency room several times thinking that I was having a heart attack and have been self-diagnosed many days. Truth be told, I am overweight, and on the inside, I know that eventually my weight would plague me. So, instead of allowing myself to be blindsided, I felt that I would just be super observant and catch the ailment before it caught me.

ELEPHANT IN THE ROOM

My mother always jokes, "You got bad genes." Between my father's side and her side, we have been plagued by it all, from diabetes to breast cancer to heart disease. This has validated my need to know what I have or at least thought I had. I can say that I hardly ever medicated myself, but I can also say I have spent hours thinking that perhaps I was coming down with a new ailment.

When I would go in for my yearly exams, I was always waiting for the other shoe to drop. I know that weight is one of the external symptoms of high blood pressure, high cholesterol, diabetes and so much more. I knew an ailment would rear its head one day. I just wanted to be prepared and not naïve like so many others.

I remember my obese-in-American-terms friend saying to me, "I am perfectly healthy and have never been sick." This was her declaration moment to say, "I am not really obese! I may have a few extra pounds, but I'm in perfect health." Well, on the inside I would giggle a little and say to myself, "We are all perfectly healthy until we're not." There are kids with perfect health until they break their arm playing, there are women with perfect health until they are diagnosed with breast cancer, and I myself was in perfect health until I needed blood-pressure medicine. You see, we are all weeks, days and moments away from our health status changing. As happy as I am that she has never had any significant health problems, I still wanted to say, "Just make sure you work to keep it that way, and if you feel something is wrong, don't be so caught up in being healthy that you over look it."

Finding out that I needed blood-pressure medicine at 30 changed things. Even though I was a lightweight hypochondriac, hearing that I needed this medicine and would need to be on it for the rest of my life changed me. The shit got real! It wasn't *them* or *her*. It was me, and at this young age, my food choices, weight and perhaps my genes lead me to this path.

As prepared as I thought I would be for this declaration by my doctor, I couldn't help but feel shocked and disappointed because I felt it was the beginning of my bad-health trajectory. This diagnosis was the single medical thing that changed the way I saw myself and my weight.

That day, I made up my mind to get weight-loss surgery. Being on the medication was the first thing that crossed my mind as to why the surgery may be necessary. I had been introduced to getting weight-loss surgery over a decade prior, but I always told the doctor, "I got this," believing that I had my weight under control. Plus, I wanted babies, and nothing I read confirmed that the surgery would not affect my ability to have a healthy pregnancy. I had been fighting the idea of surgery because it also made me feel like if I succumbed to it, officially I was a failure and a "happy big girl" fraud. How could someone educated, goal oriented, and confident not handle losing some pounds on her own? That was the thought behind this failure, and of course my soul was defined by being a happy big girl. I loved me and my thickness. I dressed cute, I had plenty of friends and could get men, and I was happy, right? But here I was in my early 30s and already beginning a blood-pressure regimen, and that is not what I wanted to continue. I knew the surgery would not be a miracle, but I knew it may be my only opportunity to reshape my health and my body. So, maybe I wasn't just worried for no reason, a hypochondriac, but in fact I was worried because I knew deep inside that my weight was the reason.

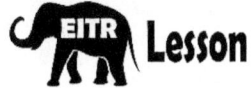 **Lesson**

Sometimes you can be happy and like who you are, but there are times when you have to make decisions bigger than the here and now. You may wrestle with the ideas of the loyalty to the self-image you created, but the only real image is a lasting one. If you succumb to poor health, you certainly may lose your confidence and maybe even your life. So, you may just have to make the biggest decision to choose you, with a little help. For me this was weight-loss surgery.

Elephant 19

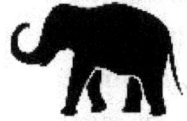

The Decision

ELEPHANT IN THE ROOM

I had thought about it for years. It had been ten years to be exact. It started with my primary care doctor years ago. I was taking prescription weight loss pills and the doctor said have you *ever* considered weight-loss surgery? Of course, my thoughts went to Al Roker and all the people who were bed ridden who had to seek surgery just to not be a prisoner in their home. But most important I thought about it as me giving up and admitting that I, Sharita Shelby, the strong, driven person, just couldn't win and get her weight under control. The thought of the surgery plagued me. I mentioned it to a few friends and my family, and at that time they said, "You don't need that!" Even though I knew it may be a good idea for me, I was scared and didn't want to look weak. Besides, I wanted to marry and have children. I was only 24, and I couldn't risk the possibility of complications. I admit, I did some research and even called my insurance, but I was glad when they said they didn't cover it because now I had an excuse that was not my own - not to have to make the choice.

Well it was ten years and about fifty pounds later. I looked at some pictures of myself on our family vacation, and I just didn't feel pretty or photogenic, as people have called me and how I self-identified. No matter at what angle I held the camera, I smiled, and my double chin was there, and I just felt fat. Not the confident big girl that I always felt I was. I knew in these moments that it was finally time. I had also been placed on blood-pressure pills at 30 years old, and that was not okay with me. This revelation began on my trip, a seven-day cruise through Cozumel, Honduras and other ports of call, in July.

So, I began to talk to my new primary care physician and she said, "I think this would be good for you. You have to lose weight, or your health will progressively get worse and you will die."

This sank in immediately. I left that appointment and immediately joined the weight-management program at the YMCA because I knew this journey had to begin now. I knew I needed more information about weight-loss surgery. That November our health-care agent at work came out to discuss our new healthcare plan, and she said weight-loss surgery was covered. Of course, the thought that this potential life-enhancing procedure could be covered by insurance was exciting, but I didn't want to get too excited or too fearful until I knew if this could happen for me.

My doctor gave me a referral to a doctor who performed the surgery, and I walked in with a plan. I wanted the least invasive surgery because I felt that it

ELEPHANT IN THE ROOM

would come with the least amount of criticism. I was an educated woman who read the reviews, studied YouTube, and had heard all the advice possible from family and friends. Besides, I was a big girl who wanted to stay true to my creed, so even though I would get surgery, I would still be plus size, and that meant I was cool and not a sellout. I walked in and to my utter shock, the doctor said, "Ms. Shelby, I will do what you ask, but the least invasive surgery"—or what I thought was the least invasive— "is not what is best for you. The results will not be what you are expecting, and I don't want you to come back later and ask why I allowed you to do this when I as your surgeon knew better."

I will admit I was frozen on the doctors table. I hadn't even considered gastric bypass surgery! I continued to sit there as he talked about the procedure, the average weight loss, and blah, blah, blah. I was shocked, I was hurt and embarrassed that I had allowed myself to get there. But I did, but I didn't! I had been working out for years. I had been on Atkins and the cabbage diet. I'd been to Slimmer Image and even Jenny Craig. I had even lost 15 pounds during the biggest loser at work. How was I the 33-year-old that needed this extensive weight-loss surgery? I can't say how I got there, but I was there, and this was what I needed to do, and this was the time.

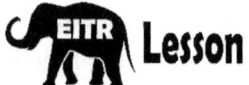 **Lesson**

I never thought my weight would get to the point that I would need the support of surgery, but it did. With all the fear in my heart, I still went through with it because ultimately it wasn't just the day-to-day battle of being obese. It was the literal war on my health. Yes! I chose the war and decided that however it turned out, it was my opportunity to choose me and start a new journey to be the best me, just a different edition.

Elephant 20

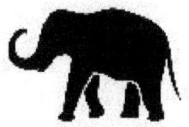

Still Big: The Post surgery Challenge

ELEPHANT IN THE ROOM

The journey of weight-loss surgery has been like a tunnel into to the unknown, and not only is it dark but it is lonely. Ninety-five percent of the people around you have no idea what you're going through. You are feeling something different within your body. You are full quicker, your shape begins to transform right in front of your very eyes, and your mind just can't catch up. The naysayers have begun their commentary, and the supporters don't know what to say. Despite your struggle to formulate "the answer and response" to their questions and your decision, the truth is, you really don't know much about your path because it is your first time on it. You have a group of your old heavy friends who felt you sold out, *and* you get your new "gym" friends who dote that they "just exercise and eat right" because they only value the "natural way" to lose weight. Then, you get with the group that never met anybody who ever had weight-loss surgery, so they skate back in forth between "You go, girl" and "You're starting to look funny. You don't wanna be the big-head-skinny-body girl." There are so many comments, but I was struggling to even give my voice to this very personal experience.

It has been since September 2013, and I can say that I am proud to have lost over one hundred pounds. To most that is like a person, and to me it was part of who I was. I am excited to finally shop in regular stores and to not have a double chin staring back at me, but it is also a world of being lost to the person and this body that you see.

All you hear from others is, "Girl, I would love to be buying smaller clothes." To them there is no struggle. "Just buy more clothes!"

These comments flow so freely, as if my life hadn't changed and isn't still changing. When I look in the mirror, I know me, but there is a part of me that misses seeing the chubby-faced girl. See, I had grown a confidence for that girl. I was the girl who prided herself and represented for the big girls. I prided myself on being a big girl with class, style and a damn good girdle! My self-empowerment came from deciding that I would represent "us," and now, things were changing. I was much smaller than I was, but to the world I'm still fat! How is that? At moments, I walk around with my head held high, like, "Look what I did!" but to them I still wear an 18, and that's still not enough! At times, you stand paralyzed at the sight that you are a size 18, when you used to squeeze in some people's 28s. Size is the number in your clothes, but it doesn't come with a mind-set to

ELEPHANT IN THE ROOM

define your body. As women we all know, in one single shopping trip, you can fit three different sizes. You are not sure whether to celebrate the lowest number or jump into an extreme diet from the highest number. This same feeling is what it feels like when you lose so much weight but the number on your tag is still "plus size." The psychological part of this life change starts to surpass the physical.

You see, once you are above a size 12, you are in the world of shopping on the other side of the store, the "special section." And as a bariatric surgery recipient, I prayed for the day that I could slide to the other side freely and pick out just what I wanted. Yes, I wanted to lose weight in numbers and be taken off my blood-pressure medication, but I also really wanted to know, for once, what the other side of life felt like. Losing all this weight and still being plus sized is a challenge in my mind. Mysteriously, I feel that now it is still not enough. It is almost like being given a scoop of confidence and someone saying, "No, you just need half a scoop."

The results of weight-loss surgery vary from person to person. My doctor reviewed this prior to the surgery, but he also stated that if you do what you need to, you will get the desired weight-loss results.

ELEPHANT IN THE ROOM

I never wanted to be a size 6, never, but I did at least want to shop on the other side. I'm grateful for the surgery because I know it saved my life, but damn, I wasn't expecting this. I wanted to, for once, see fashion and immediately get to purchase what I like. Being plus size has been decades of finding your style within the available choices. I could never just select style, size, and color and order. In order to piece together my style, I may have to get my wear-to-work classic pieces from Lane Bryant, my size 12 shoes from the Avenue, my trendy shirt from Ashley Stewart, and my accessories from Forever 21.

I never made it to the single digits, and I'm sure I never will. But I will say that it is a challenge to put in all the work, yes, *all* the work that goes into preparing for surgery, living a bariatric lifestyle, no soda, alcohol, vitamins every day, still working out, and never getting to order my *size 12*! The Zumba, the water aerobics, the liquid diets, the throwing up, and a ton of unsolicited feedback, and here I am … still big!

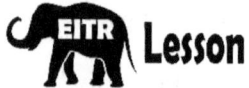 **Lesson**

Even after losing one hundred pounds and being taken off blood-pressure medication, the mental stamp placed on me by my America still resounds in my mind. It should be enough just to be healthier and of course a few sizes smaller, but the unsaid message stamped in my head is since I was not size 12 or under, I still was a second-class woman.

Elephant 21

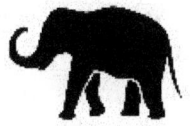

I Get an A for Acceptance

ELEPHANT IN THE ROOM

There is a single moment that you have to make the choice about yourself and the life you are meant to have. God created us in all colors, shapes and sizes. Our noses, our lips, our facial contours are all unique to us. The very things that we sometimes don't like are the very unique things that define our beauty and uniqueness. Our personality begins to be developed as young as four years old, when our sense of humor, our temperament, and our free-ness begin to be defined. These things begin to build the person we see in the mirror. But there are single moments where you look in the mirror and you decide to choose you and accept you - flaws and all. I remember there were a few defining moments that chose me, and I was willing to accept me.

The first moment was when I was around seven years old, and I thought I wanted to kill myself and my dad said, "Don't let anybody make you ever want to hurt you." I was young, but his advice made sense, and in that moment, I decided that my journey was mine. I could only be me, and even if I was the only one rooting for me, that would have to be okay. I had to step into my first moment of acceptance. I know I was a little girl, and I can't even say that I wanted to

die when I thought of killing myself. I just wanted to be missed and noticed by my mother, not because of my differences from her and other girls, but just for being the chubby little brown girl that was hers. I am not sure that I comprehended everything in that moment, but I know that I understood that there was going to be a "different journey ahead because of my weight," and I was going to have to rely more on me. As years have gone by, I have evolved more from that lesson. This was the beginning of my road to acceptance.

The next defining moment came when I was about fourteen years old. I remember looking at my girl cousins and seeing that they were smart, talented, popular, fashionable and *thin!* I noticed all the attention they received, and even though I was okay with my life because I always saw myself as different than them, I liked the image of them being well put together. I wanted to be made up, look nice, smell good and most important be sure of myself and know I could look as good as everyone else. Not only did I like the images of my cousins but many other "well put together" women, too. From that moment on, I read magazines, I studied women that I admired, I listened more in conversation about self-care and beauty routines. I accepted my version of what that would be. That was the research to create the confidence that I needed to come into my own as I began developing into a young woman.

One of the final times I remember having a self-defining and accepting moment was in college. It was my junior year, I had run for student government president of Fisk University and I lost by a reported less than fifty votes. In this moment, I felt hurt because I believed I was the best candidate and I felt that my smartness, well roundedness and love for Fisk would translate into being the leader of this institution. I felt my résumé was more than enough and my experiences with all my fellow Fiskites, peer students, would allow me to get this "position" that I wanted. But the moment I lost was a moment of acceptance and clarity for me. Here I was in the cafeteria with all my friends and the friends of my opponent, and I had to smile and be able to walk out that door with my head held high. Immediately I had to just think and accept this loss. I had to accept that this role did not define my work, my commitment, or my love for Fisk. Just maybe this position was not the position God wanted for me. I smiled in that moment, thanked all my friends, and decided to hold my head up and walk through the campus to attend class. This loss didn't mean I was a loser. It just meant that I was not appointed to this position. It was one of the moments where I can say I had to truly accept myself, and it defined who I would be as a woman.

Defining moments would come throughout this journey to almost 40 years of age. Times that stand out define moments of acceptance. And, even at this moment, I am standing amid a new acceptance of myself. My body has changed, my family does not live in the city where I reside, my jobs have changed within my career, and I am single, sitting here knowing that it is time for more acceptance. These are the moments that we all need to experience, as we exist. Nobody will accept us and love us if we don't accept ourselves. It is not saying that you're flawless, but it is saying that you are sure of all that you are and open to all that God wants you to be. You deserve an A- an A for *acceptance*.

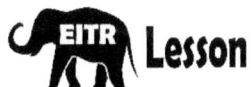# Lesson

We all have moments, but we all don't sit in the lessons of these moments. These are opportunities of awareness, and they can give definition to our path. All three of my most defining moments had little to do with my weight but more to do with

wanting more for myself and choosing how I would receive life's situations and the character I would chose to follow. Think back to times that defined you, good or bad and about all the choices you made because of them. The great news is that all of us have the opportunity to redefine our lives and create moments that validate our acceptance, and for that we all get an A!

ELEPHANT IN THE ROOM

Elephant 22

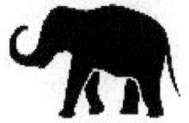

Looking to the Hills

ELEPHANT IN THE ROOM

Throughout this book you have been able to take a glimpse at my life as a plus-size woman in America, but this is the part when I get on my soapbox. In church, there is a scripture that says, "I look to the hills from which cometh my help." This chapter is called "Looking to the Hills." This simply means put your head up, straighten up your back, and walk in the life God gave you with grace and with pride. Whether you are a size 2 or a 22, it takes time to just feel good in your skin and to love your body! But do it! It amazes me how we all have a part of our body we are not happy about, and we all think we need to lose at least 15 pounds always, but yet we look at heavier women with dismay. Most of our weight gain began at just 15 pounds, but we were not prepared for life, stress, and just the mind frame needed to lose weight. We judge other women's lives before they say one word. We think that all they do is eat, that they don't want to change, and some of you have even thought of it as disgusting. Well, hell, maybe someone hurt their bodies, and they eat to make it unattractive, so no one will hurt their bodies again. Maybe after the kids it was just a slow ten pounds at a time, and they felt too far gone to change it. Or, was it just that they had been "heavy" since they were children and started to just love and accept

ELEPHANT IN THE ROOM

the skin they were in, like me? It is not that we don't notice our size, but we have grown to love and dress our bodies cute and move forward. At times, I purposely didn't diet because I was too tired to worry about it, and I was gonna eat exactly what I wanted. Ever so often I wanted to escape the day-to-day pressure of being overwhelmed with my weight-loss journey.

Before you judge me, your daughter, friend, sister, cousin or even yourself, know that life is a journey and to have the world get to notice your wrong or struggle every day is challenging. A gambler can lose his money at a casino, and no one would ever know. Even an alcoholic can get drunk and fall out and people say, "Whoa! That was a crazy night!" not acknowledging the addiction, and still no one would ever know. People even get to walk around using illegal drugs, and still no one would ever know. But everyone can see your size and feel that they have the right to weigh in. They get to look at you when they think you must be in the wrong store. They get to brag about their diet and exercise routines as if you haven't tried it ever. They post "I don't like big girls" as a status on social media. The world gets to judge us every day and get away with it. I am blessed to know that I am more than my body. I am brains, wit, charm, a Christian, a sister, a friend, and God's child, but the world is cruel, so I say to all, look to the hills from which cometh your help. Our only help comes from God!

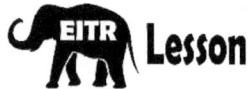 **Lesson**

In our permanent home in heaven, I believe that we are our purest self, all our imperfections are exactly our perfections. We are young at heart. While on earth we can't spend so much time on the exterior of where our souls reside. We should take a deeper look into people, challenge their thoughts, and understand their hearts. Be patient with their story and understanding to their truth because it is merely their life from their perspective. The elephant in the room is not weight. The elephant in the room is love and purity. We are not afraid to judge weight and appearance, but we are afraid to love what is not like us - to overlook the delicate imperfections. Let's not be afraid to talk about what is there instead of spending so much time focusing on only what the naked eye can see in all of us.

ELEPHANT IN THE ROOM

We were all born with love and acceptance, but when we realized we saw our first elephant, we began to alter our view, change our spirit, and doubt our hearts as we become adults. The only elephant in this room is you and me.

Elephant 23

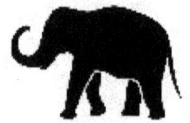

I Come as One, but I Stand as Ten Thousand

ELEPHANT IN THE ROOM

When Oprah and Maya Angelou said this, I am sure there was a deeper meaning. It even is deeply felt for me because it captures exactly the way I feel as Miss Plus-Sized America. I do believe the title exists, so I better watch calling myself that, but this resonates for the young girl that I was and all the heavy young girls that are out there.

We all will have our moment when we become okay with who we are and how we want to be portrayed. For me, I decided that I would be a diva. I wanted to be intentional about fashion, I appreciated makeup, and most important I would walk with confidence. I would look at magazines and read about skin, makeup and clothes. I would watch women who I felt were beautiful and make an effort to be similar. Of course, this was a challenge due to the limits of the clothing that was available to me, but I was determined that I would be the best me that I could be.

To all the girls who are beautiful on the inside and just waiting for the outside to catch up, I say just keep going. It's only a matter of time before you are the diva. I despised the fact for years that I thought my inside was so good but that my outside was not as flawless and acceptable. I honored my parents. I went to church. I was a good friend. I made good grades. I tried to be kind to others and respect adults. I could make you laugh, and I could befriend the guys, but I just had to do it in a size XL, 18/20, 22/24.

From starting with my cousins in mind, I learned very quickly that I couldn't use them as an example because they weren't like me, so I quit looking to them. I thought I would just start with me. For these years I have stood just as one, but as I have matriculated through life's journey, I realize that I stand as ten thousand. I represent more than ten thousand women that carry weight but also carry the load of the criticism and sometimes shame, but most important just understanding and accepting being plus size in a small-person world. This is our life, and here I stand!

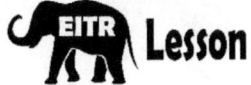 **Lesson**

Stand for yourself! Stand for others! Stand for love. At the end of the day, we are more similar than different. Therefore, don't let your weight be anyone's elephant. Let's talk about it. Laugh about it. Cry about it, and embrace it. If change is on the menu, then order it. If not, stand as one, as you too, will represent ten thousand.

ELEPHANT IN THE ROOM

ELEPHANT IN THE ROOM

ELEPHANT IN THE ROOM

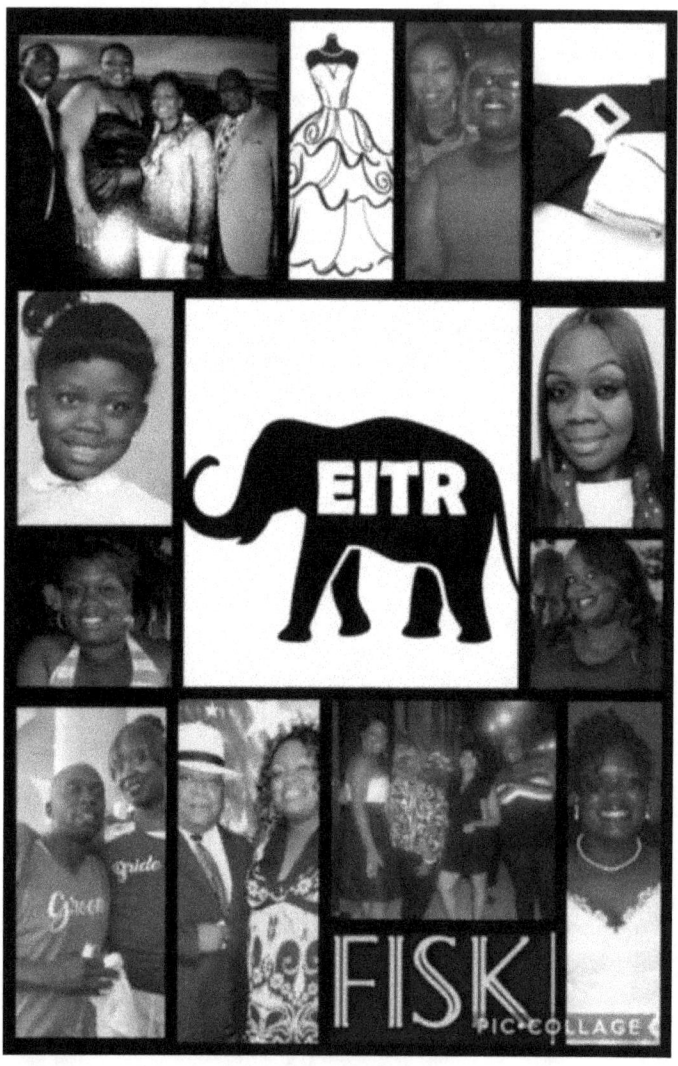

ELEPHANT IN THE ROOM

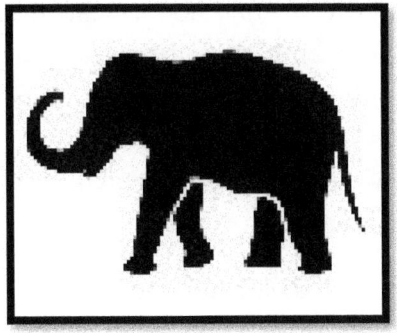

Tackling the Elephant

You have heard about my Elephants. My experiences that were often swept under the rug, some told straight to my face, others simply implied. These experiences shaped my being and my confidence. No one single incident could have done this alone. I had to learn and grow in child hood, create my place in high school, leave my mark in college and then just some good old fashioned adulting in more recent years. If there is an elephant experience that you share with me or you have your own, you must tackle them.

- Tackling the elephants sometimes, is a quiet internal conversation about how something made you feel, identifying, if you like the feeling, and then deciding how to deal with it in the future.

- Tackling is sometimes standing up to a person telling them you are not interested in their unsolicited feedback.

- Tackling is sometimes laughing and moving on.

ELEPHANT IN THE ROOM

- Tackling is sometimes surrounding yourself with people that love you and letting their love shield you from the hurts of others.

- Tackling is sometimes-researching looks, styles, lipsticks and clothes that resonate with your inner self.

- Tackling can even mean just sitting silently.

However, you choose to tackle, know you must tackle the elephant. Yes, it seems so big and powerful, but with a game plan and a steady/confident mind, you are capable of anything. There should be nothing in the world people should be able to do or say that you have not already heard, thought about or have your armor to tackle. That is where your power lies.

Let your journey be full of your ideas, so even if you fail, you begin to have a confidence in your own voice and choices. How would you ever learn your voice if you never had to go through things to help find it? My defining moments are moments that I chose to honor my voice or thoughts in spite of opposition. I could have walked away from those moment with my head down, second guessing my looks , or feeling I wasn't worthy of life ,But I chose to figure out the lesson, know that I was more than

ELEPHANT IN THE ROOM

the comments, and know that one day, I would arrive at being just the person I was supposed to be . Many sheep are dressed in elephants clothing. They use their perceived power to talk about you, make you feel less, and point out your flaws all to cover up the real elephant, that they are insecure and unsure of themselves.

Elephant in the Room is my journey, my stories, my insight, my beliefs but I challenge you to be aware of your story, your voice and create your ways to tackle your elephants!

ELEPHANT IN THE ROOM

ELEPHANT IN THE ROOM

ELEPHANT IN THE ROOM

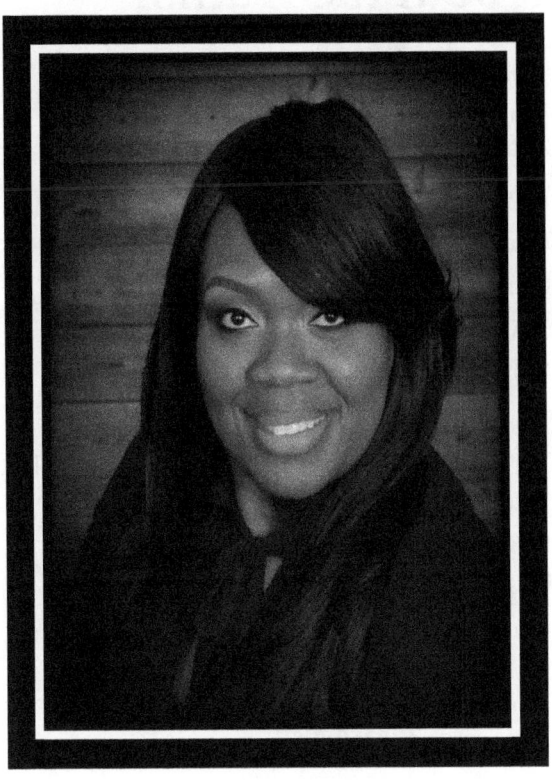

About the Author

S. Shelby is an outgoing, funny and driven woman. She has a Masters Degree in Counseling from St. Louis University and has been a Licensed Professional Counselor in Missouri and North Carolina for over a decade. She is a proud graduate of a Historically Black College, Fisk University. A member of Alpha Kappa Alpha Sorority Incorporated. She can listen to Christmas music all year around. She is a lover of self-help books and is a student of life. She is from Kansas City, Missouri, and enjoys traveling, being with friends and strengthening her voice through life experiences. She loves public speaking and empowering others. She embraces her size, her life and her gift to share with others!

Please visit:

www.eitr-sshelby.com

ELEPHANT IN THE ROOM

www.ingramcontent.com/pod-product-compliance
Lightning Source LLC
Chambersburg PA
CBHW061658040426
42446CB00010B/1793